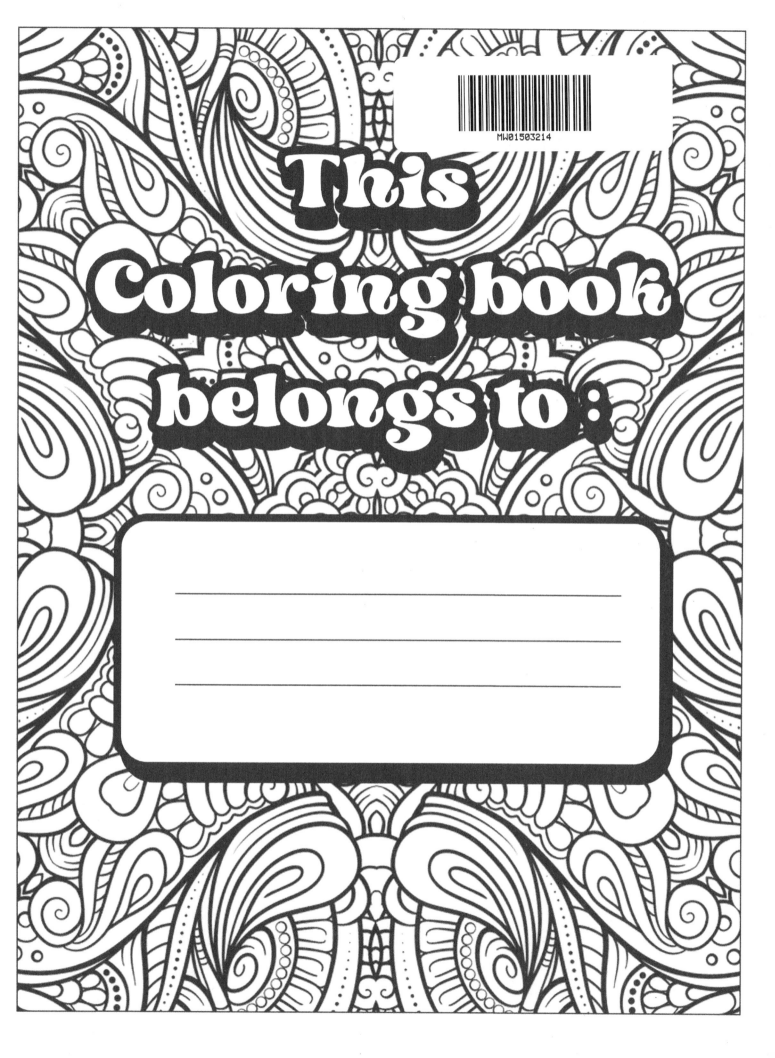

COLOR TEST PAGE

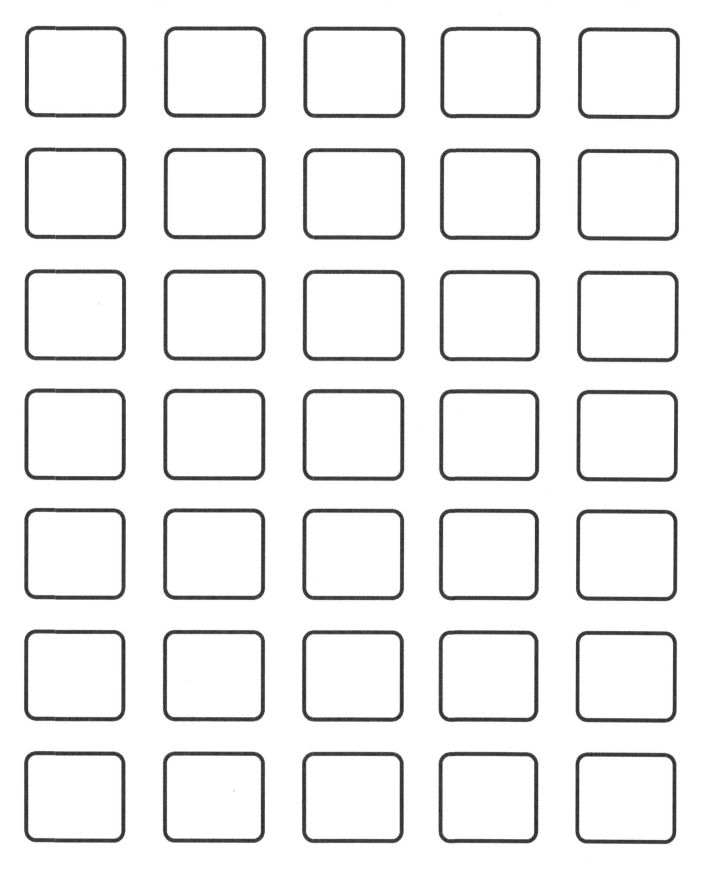

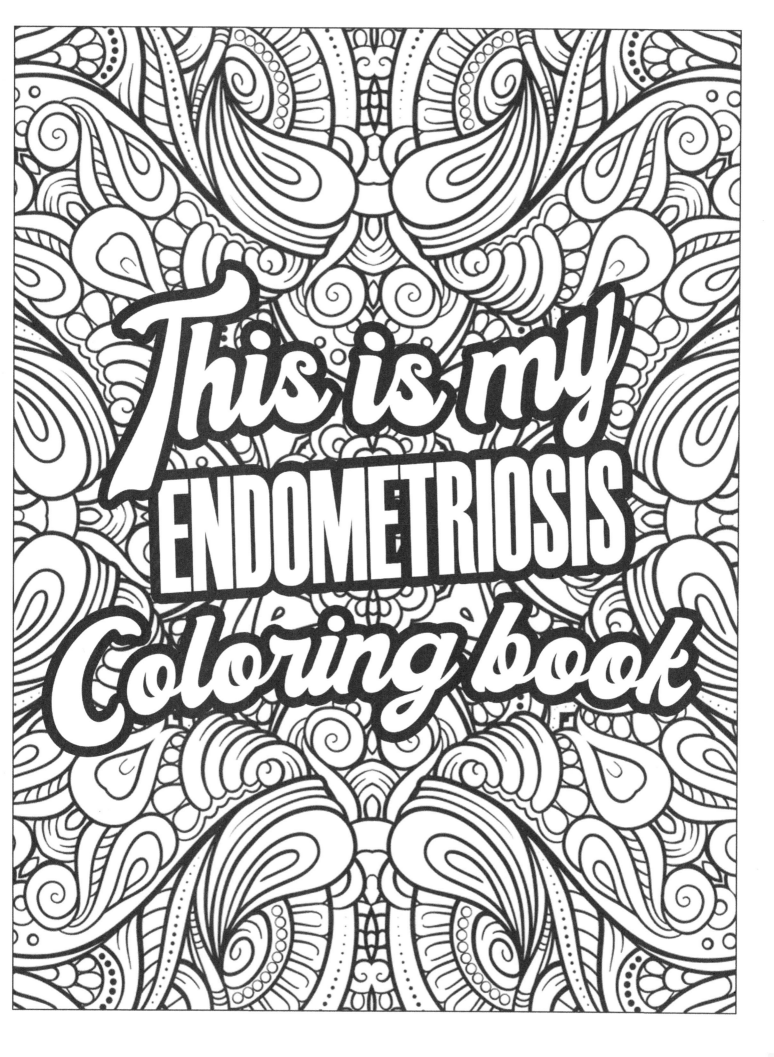

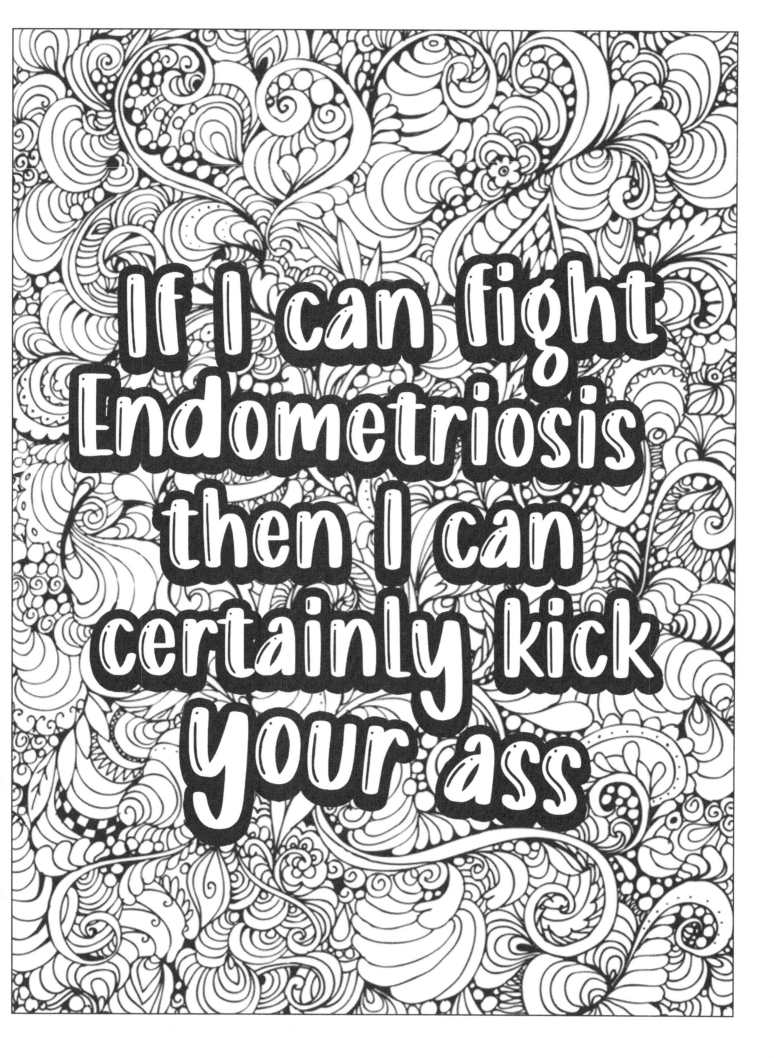

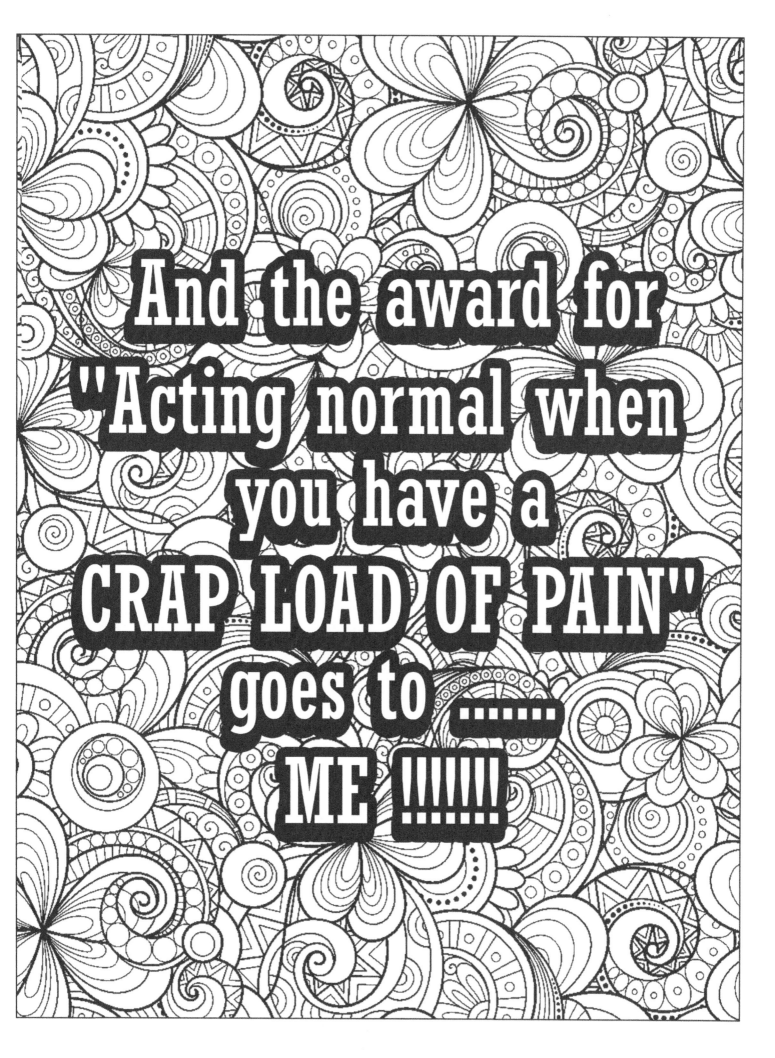

And the award for "Acting normal when you have a CRAP LOAD OF PAIN" goes to .... ME !!!!!!!

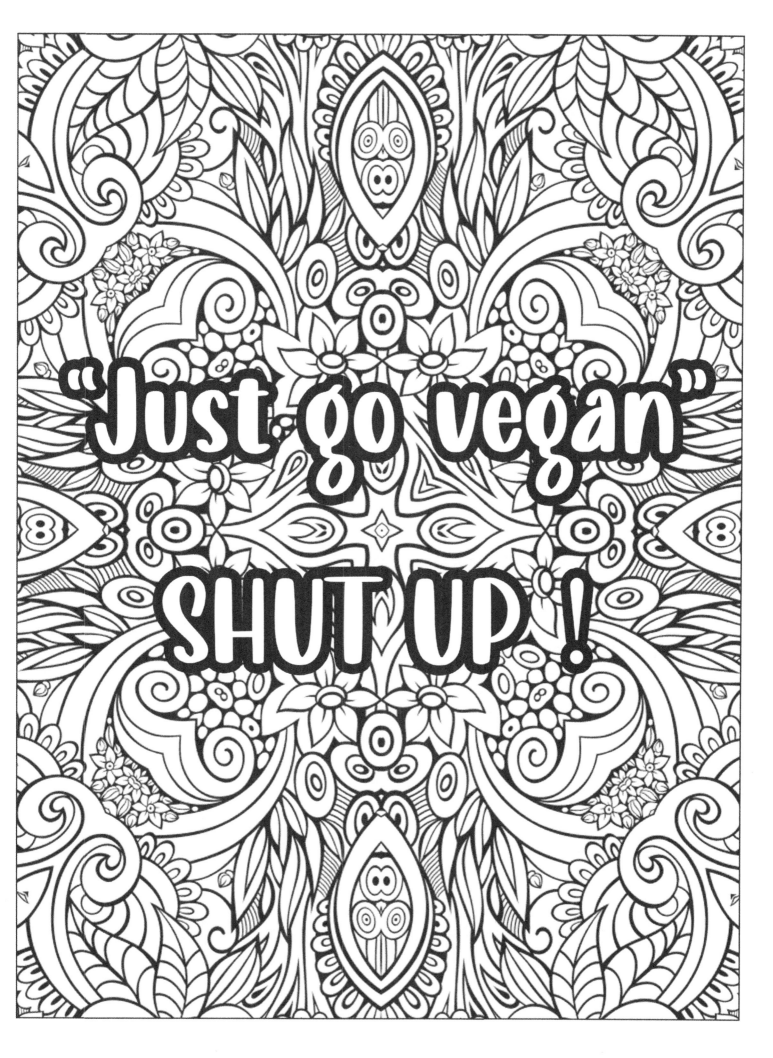

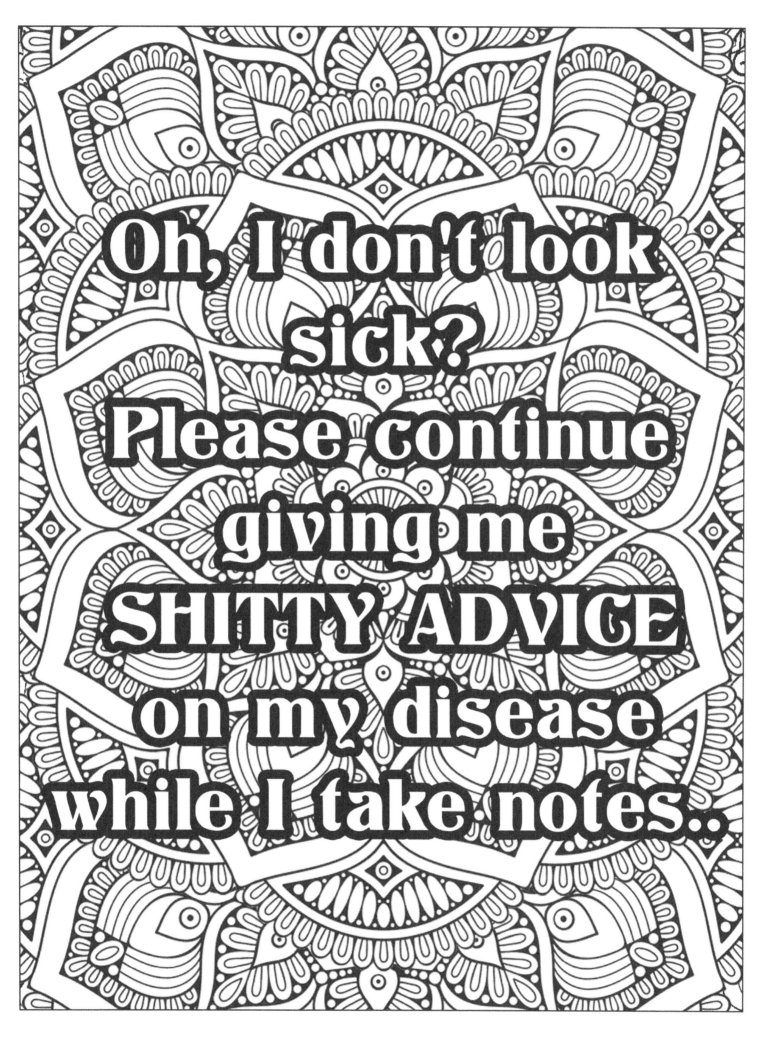

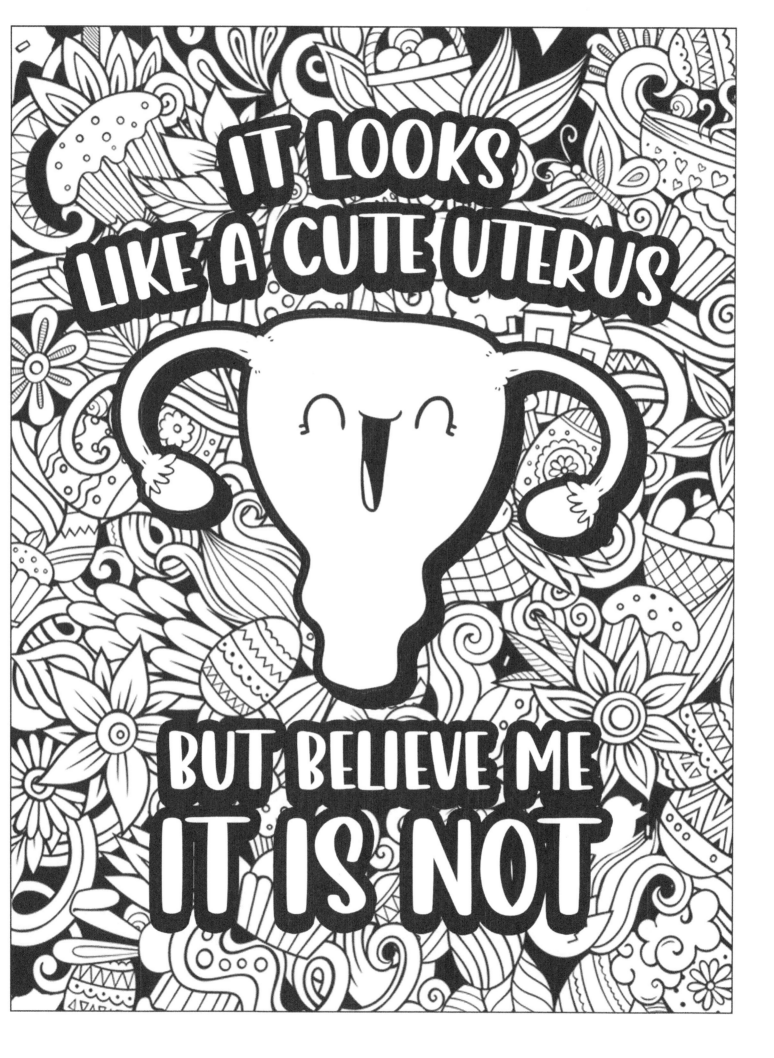

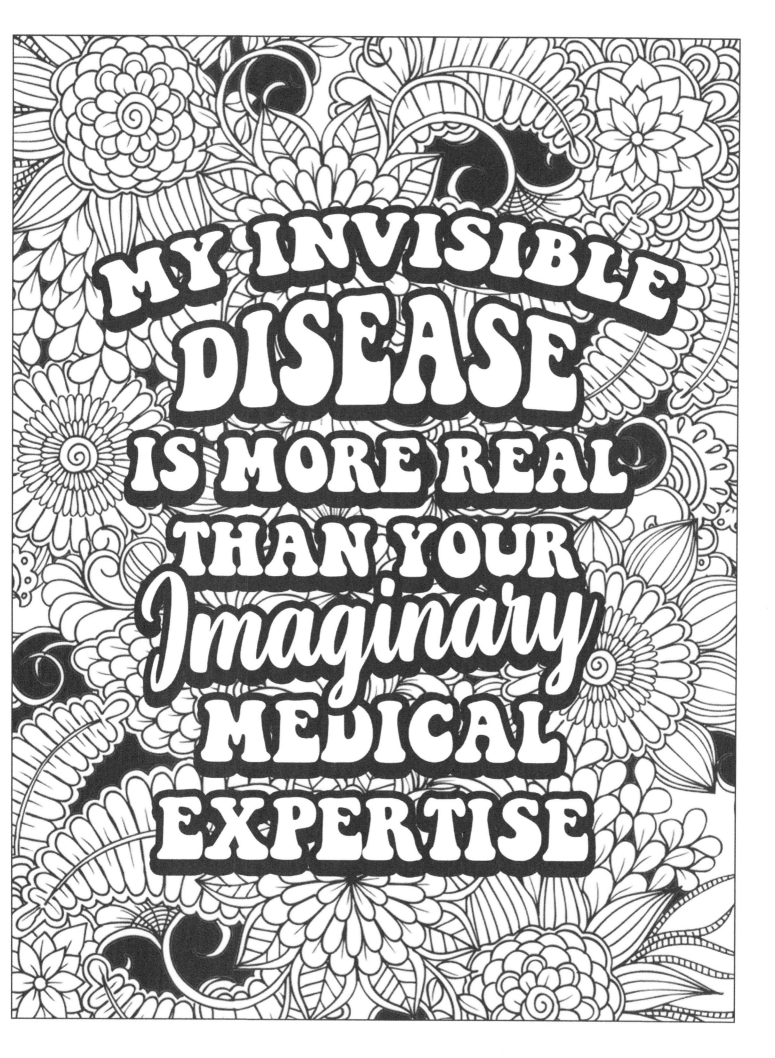

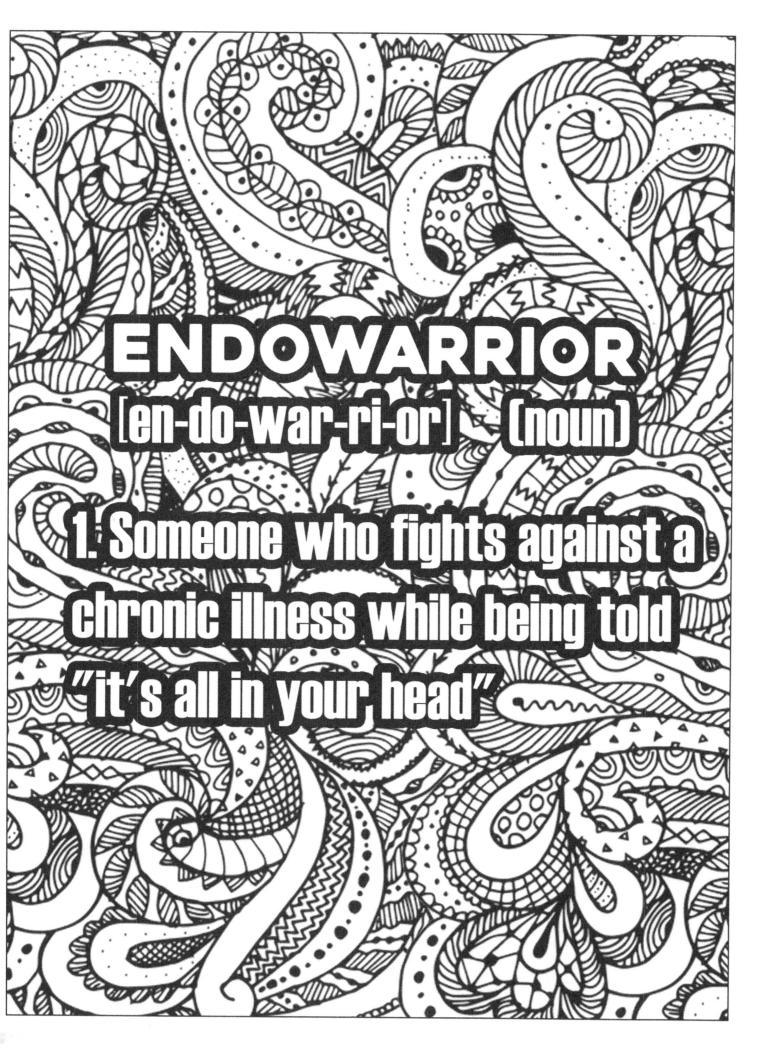

ENDOWARRIOR
[en-do-war-ri-or]   (noun)

1. Someone who fights against a chronic illness while being told "it's all in your head"

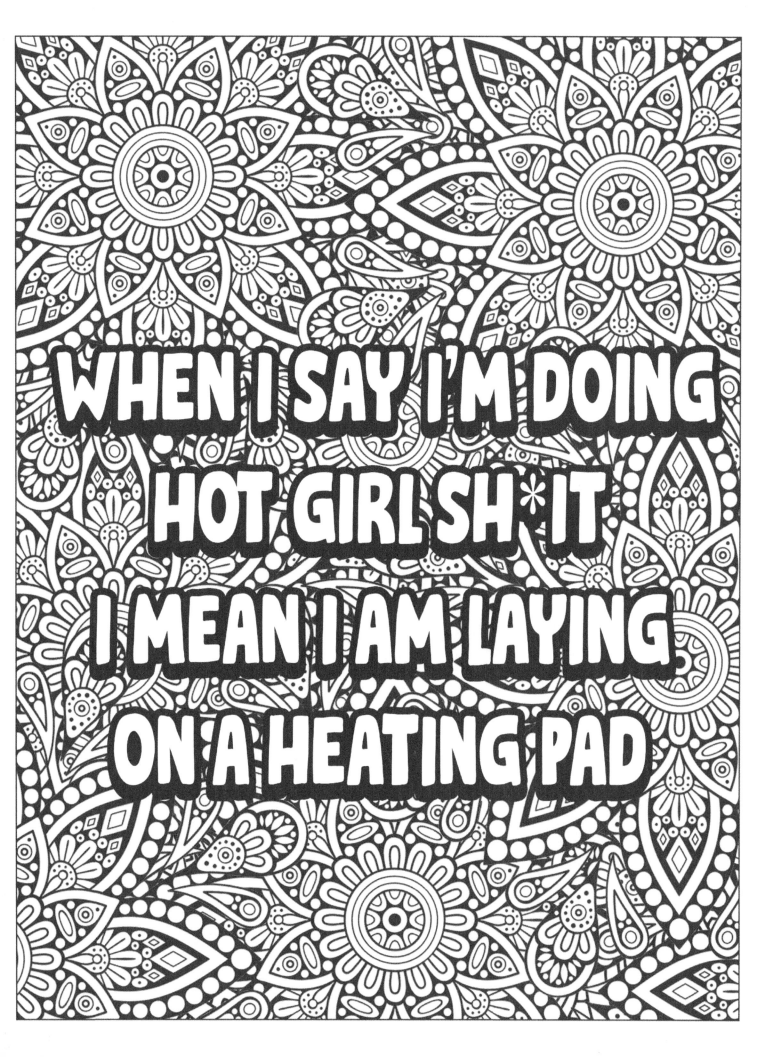

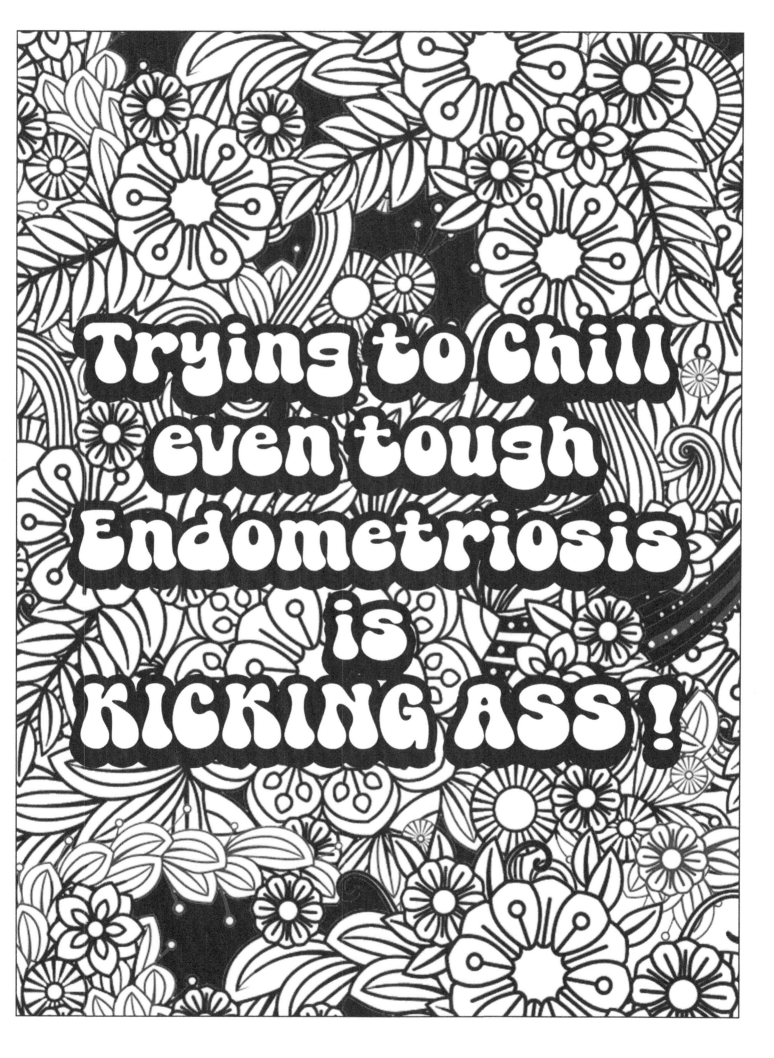

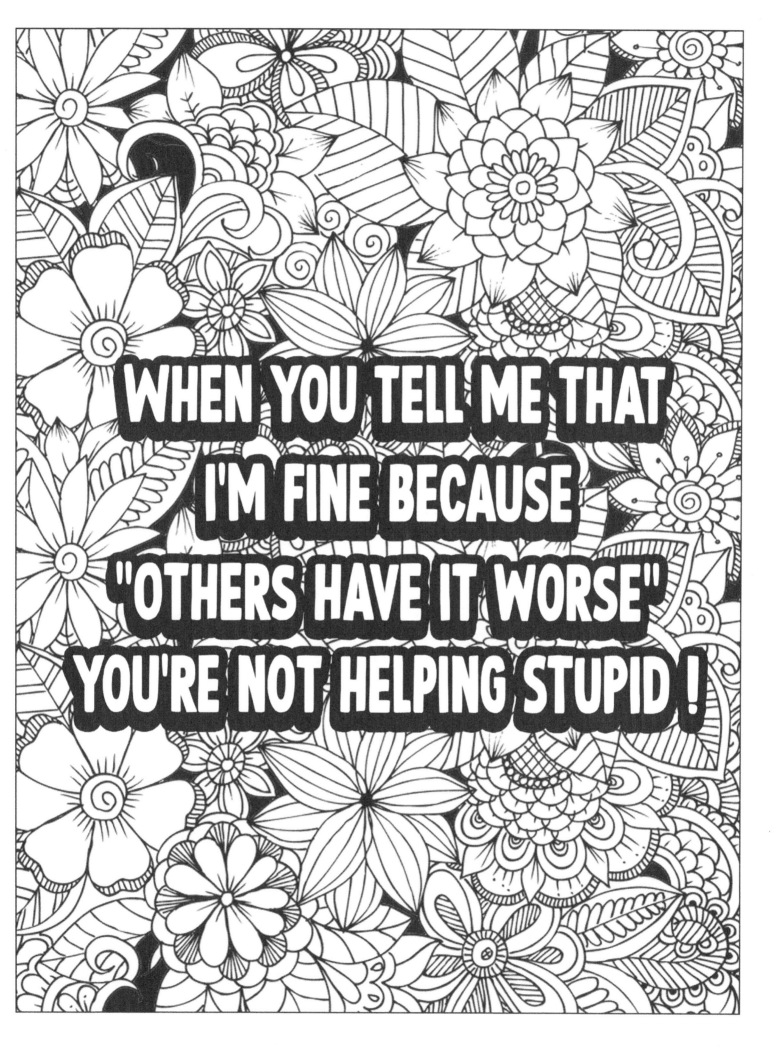

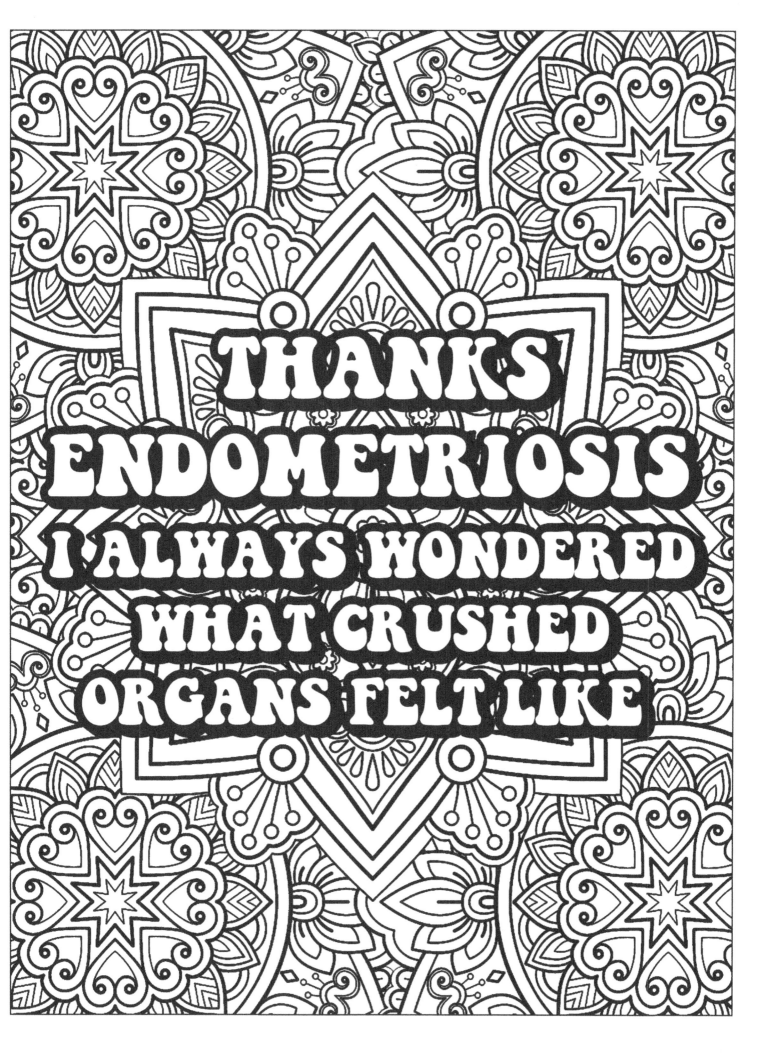

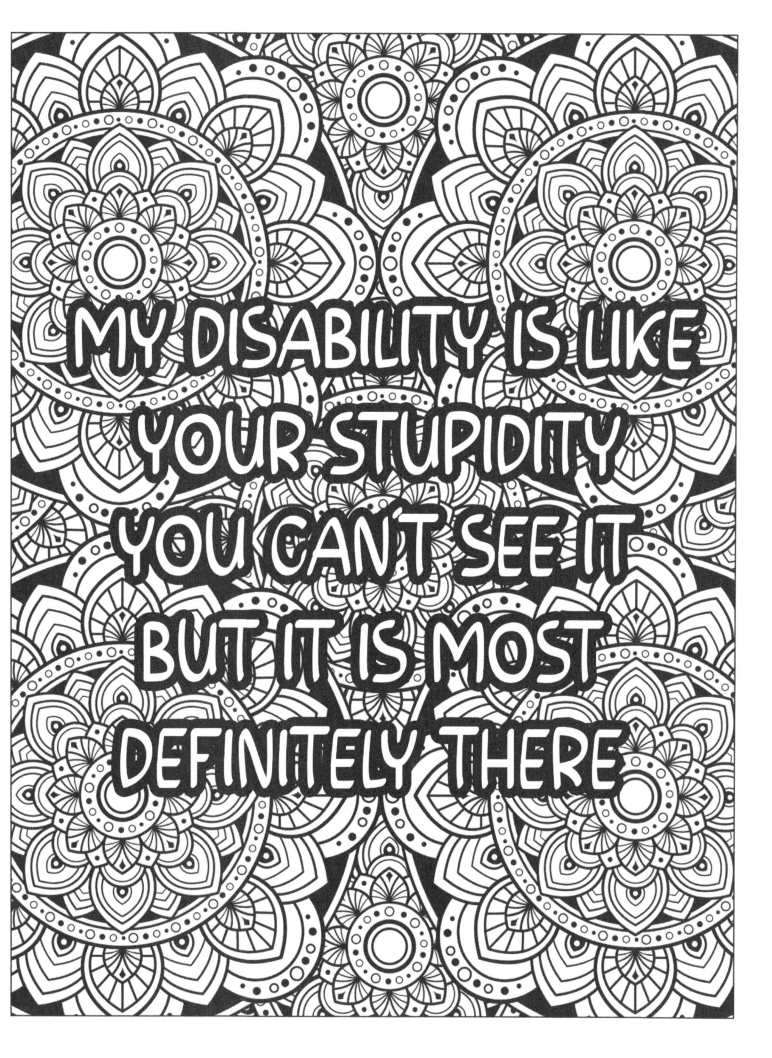

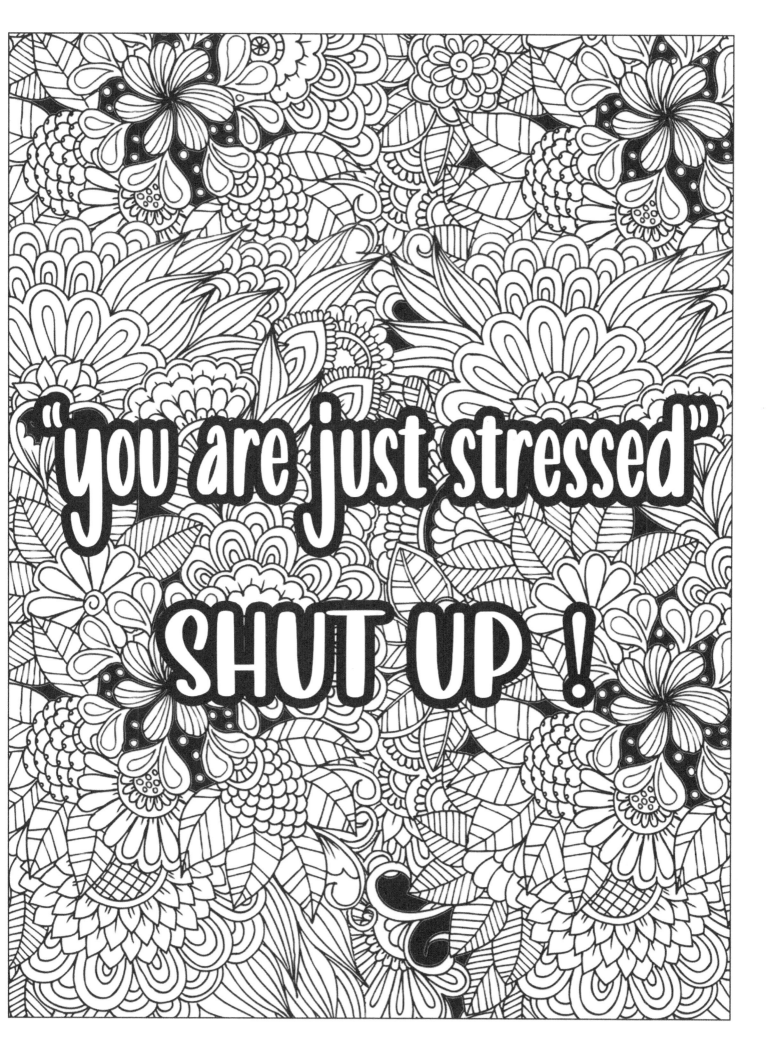

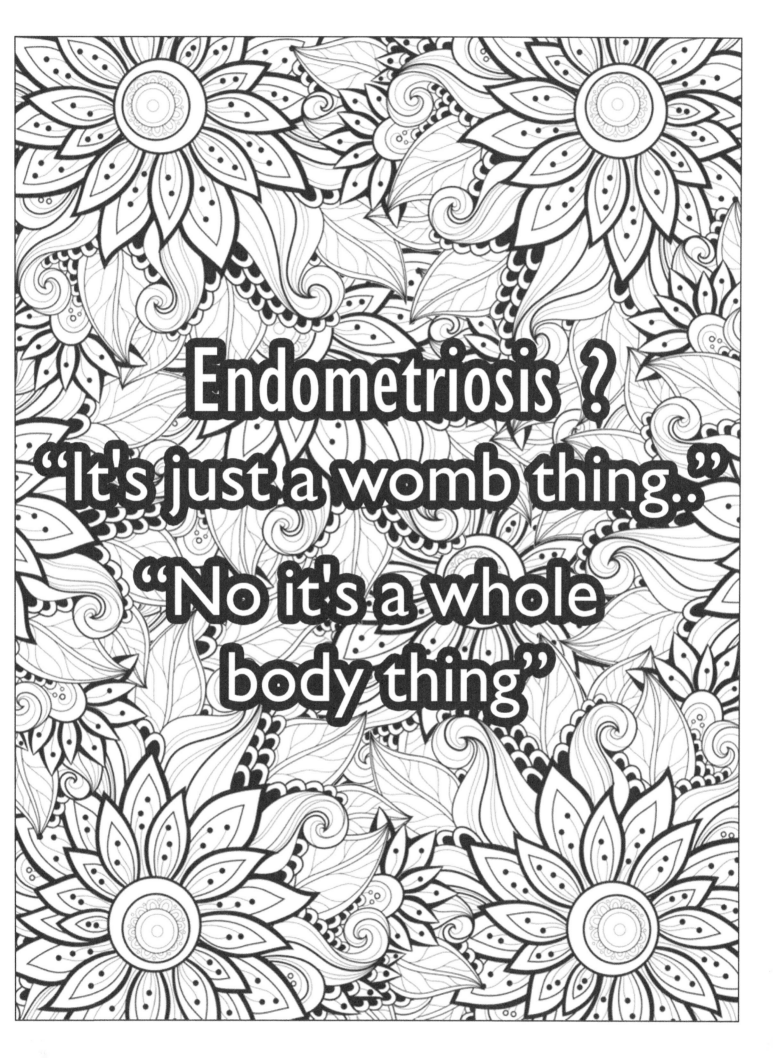

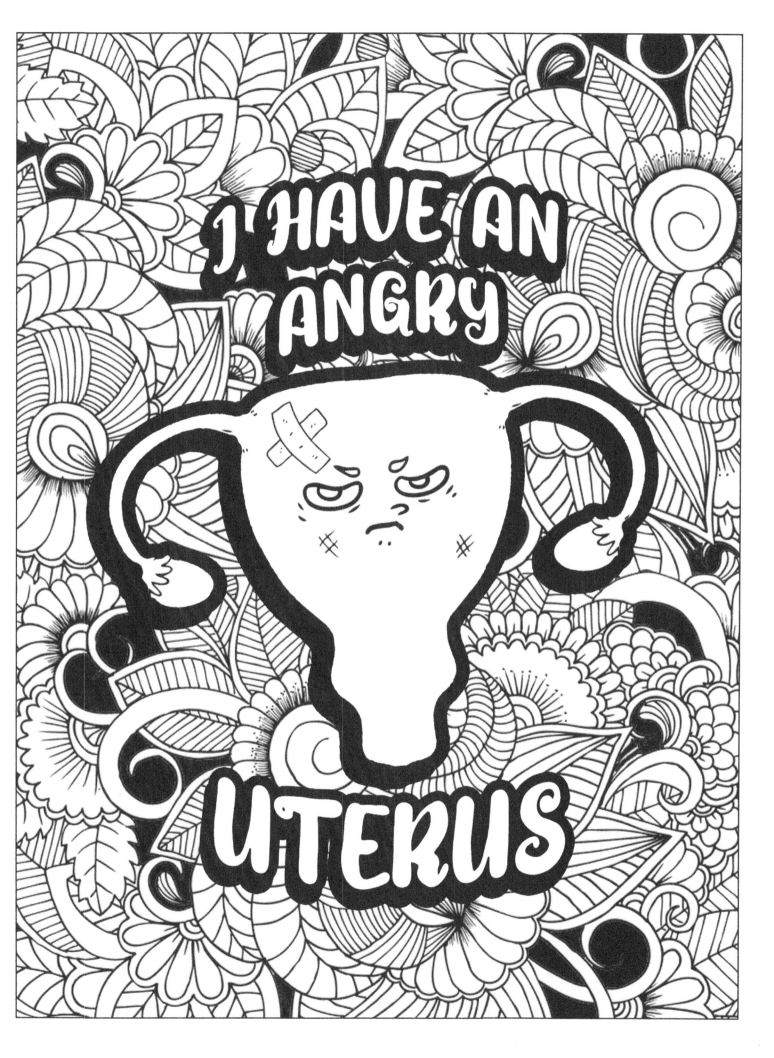

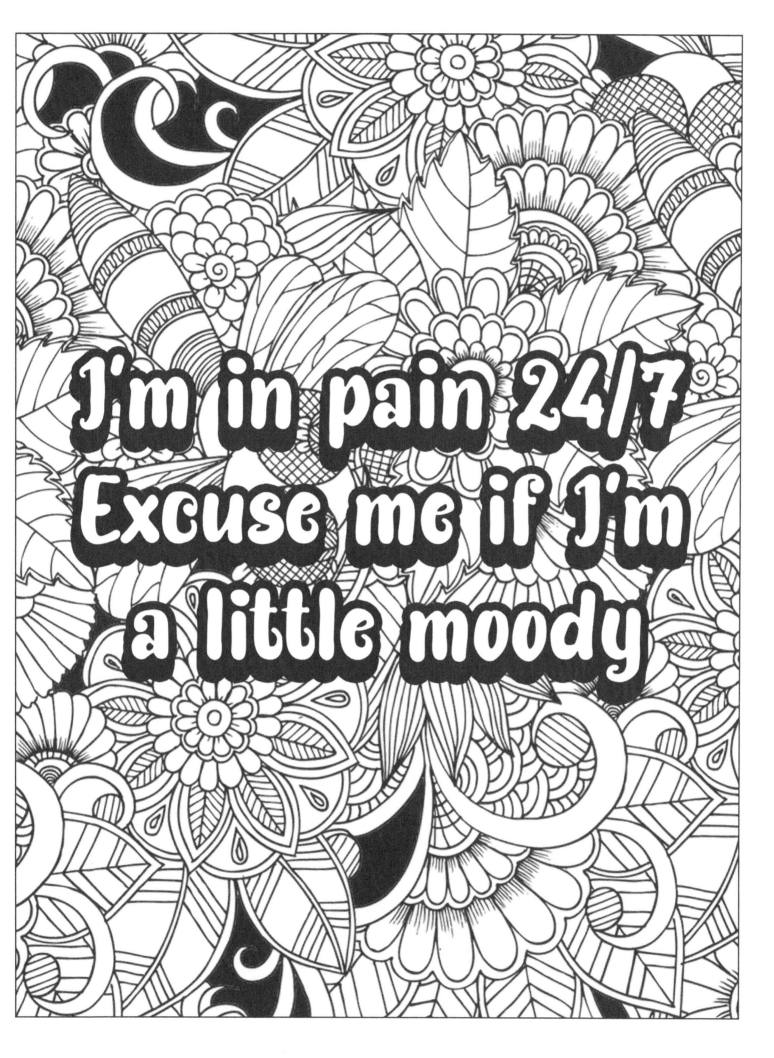

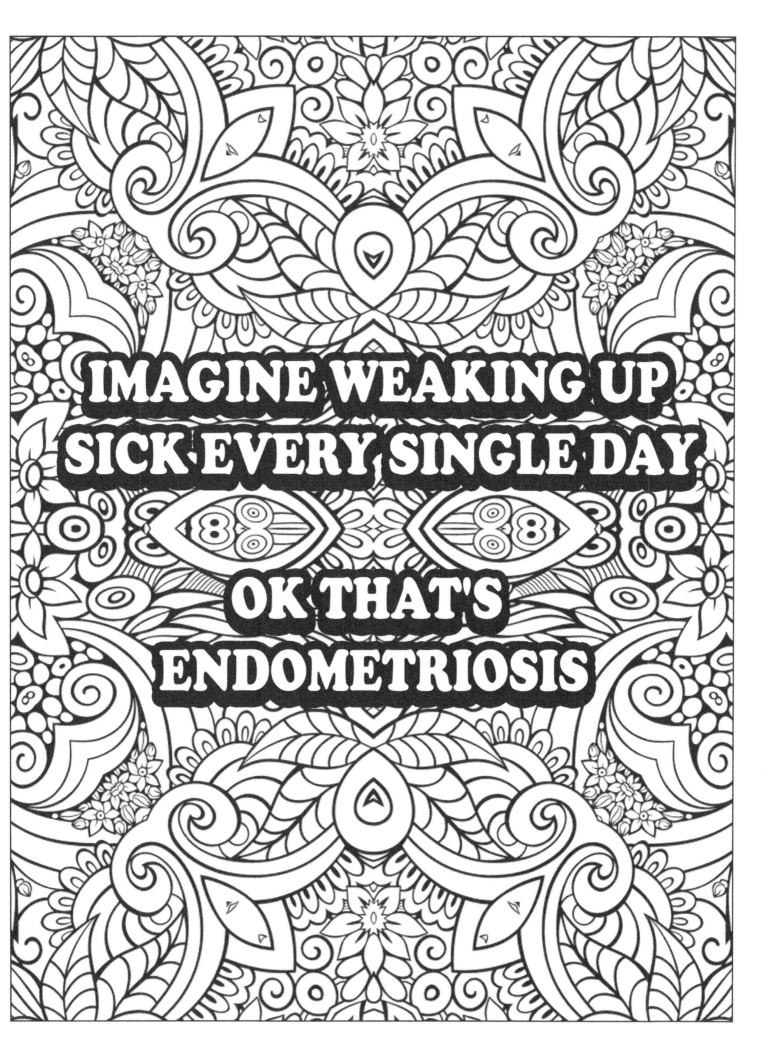

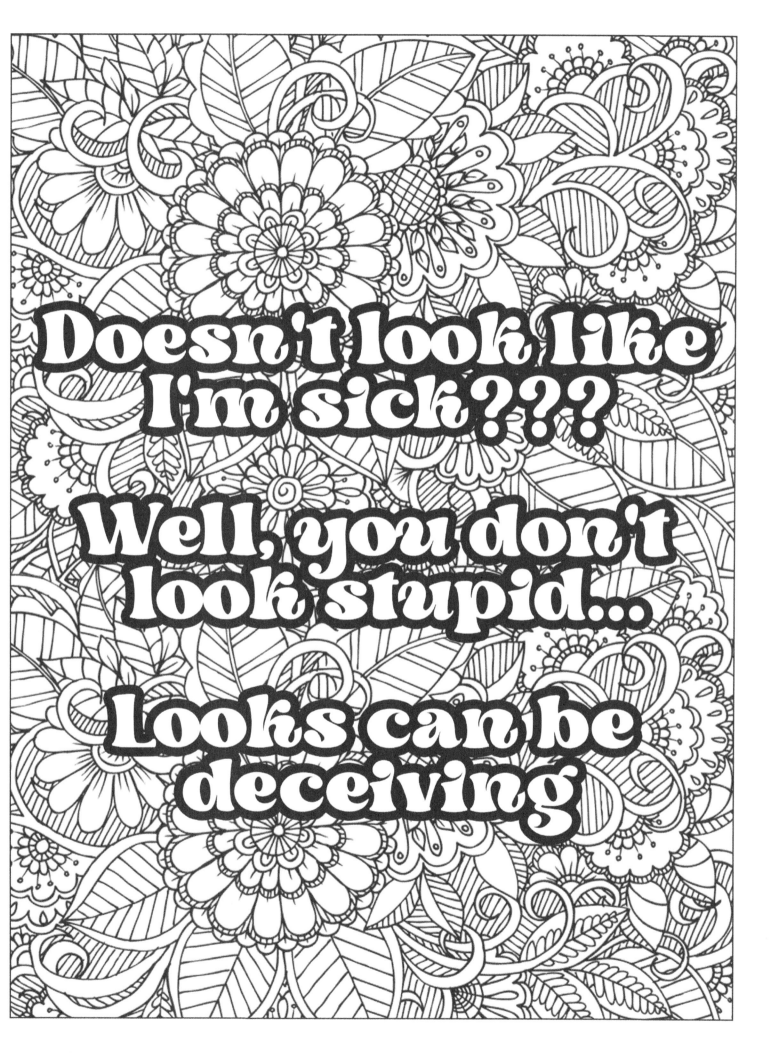

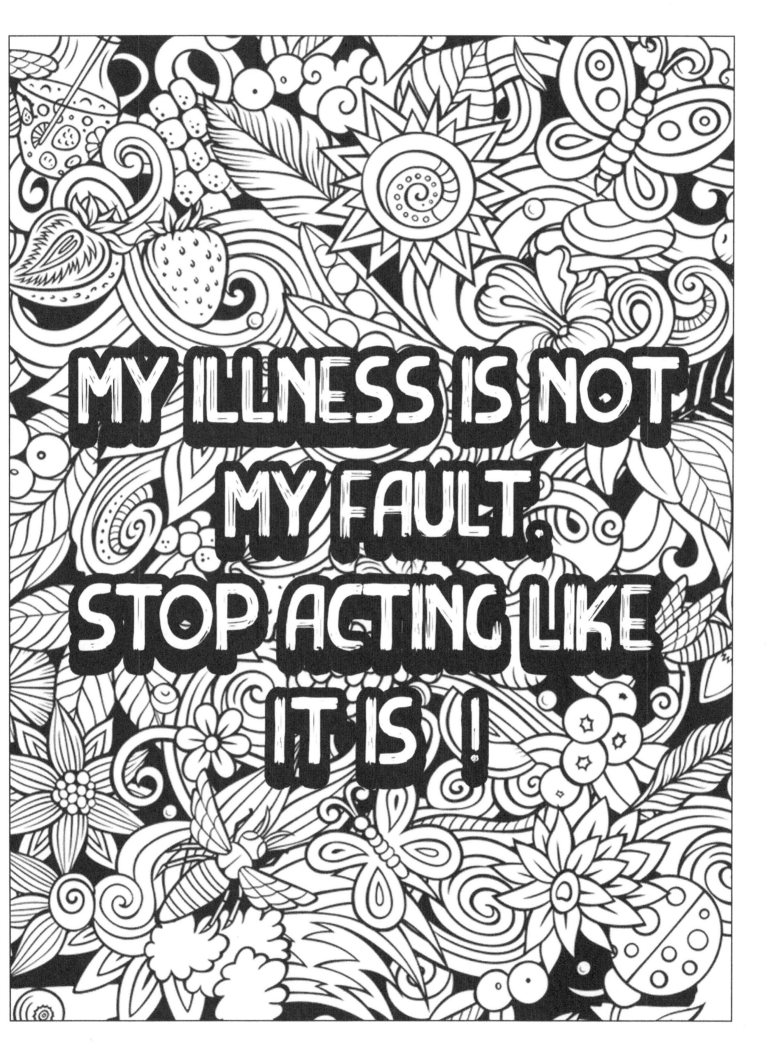

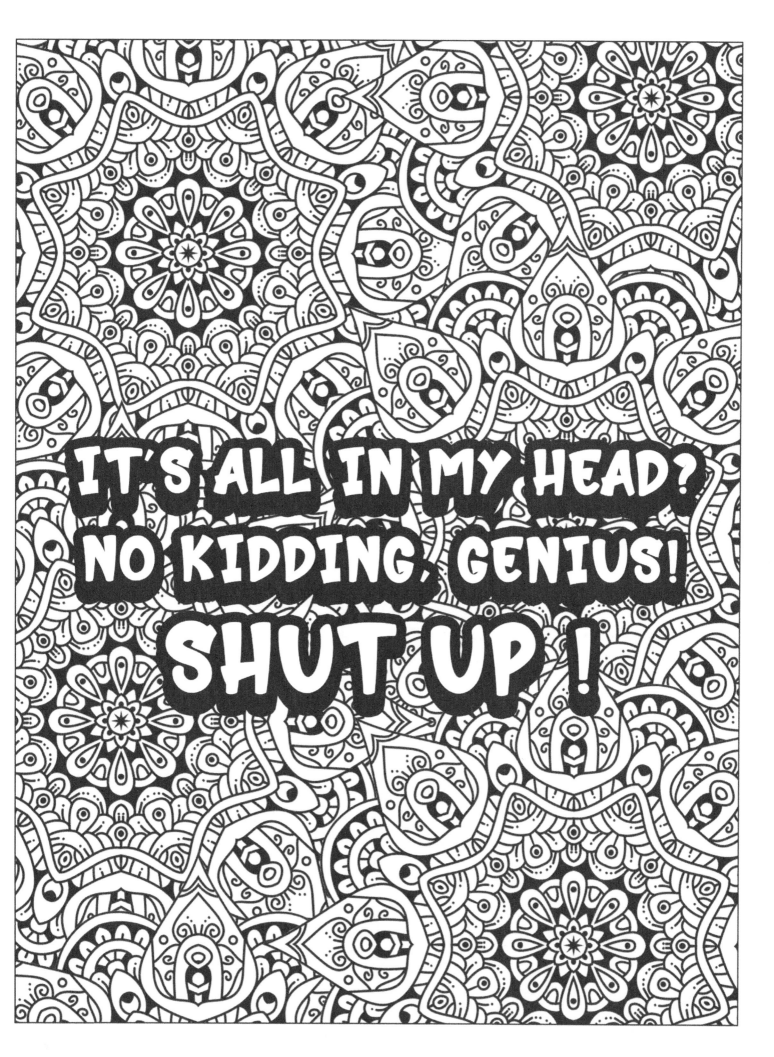

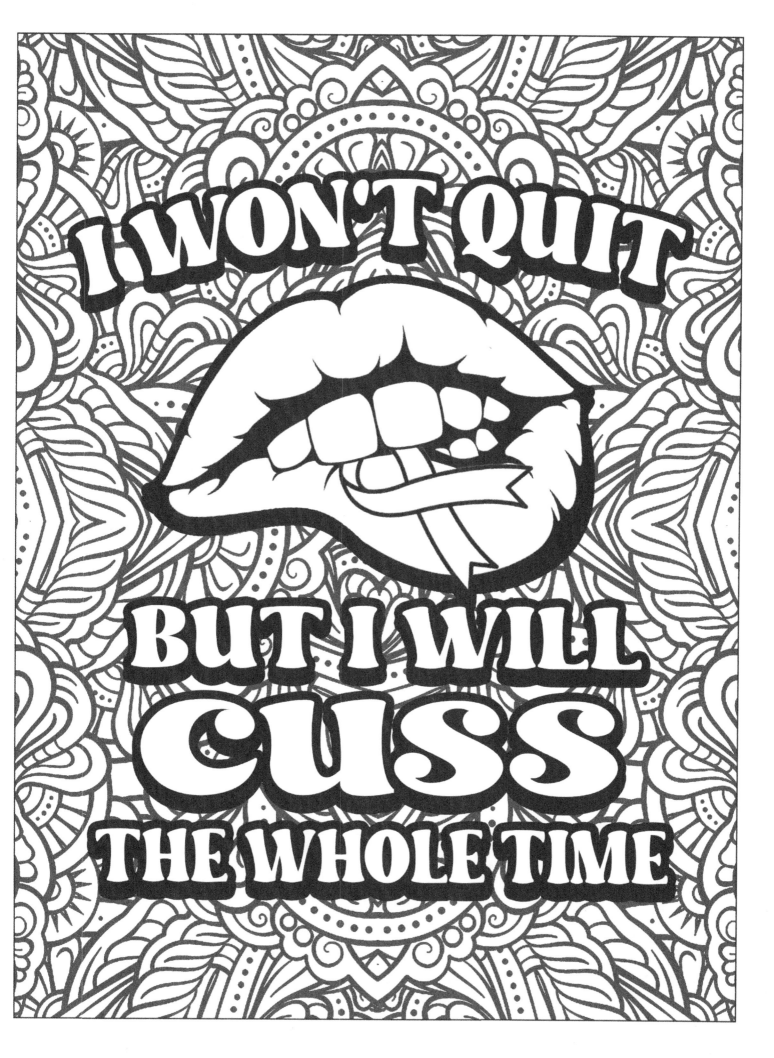

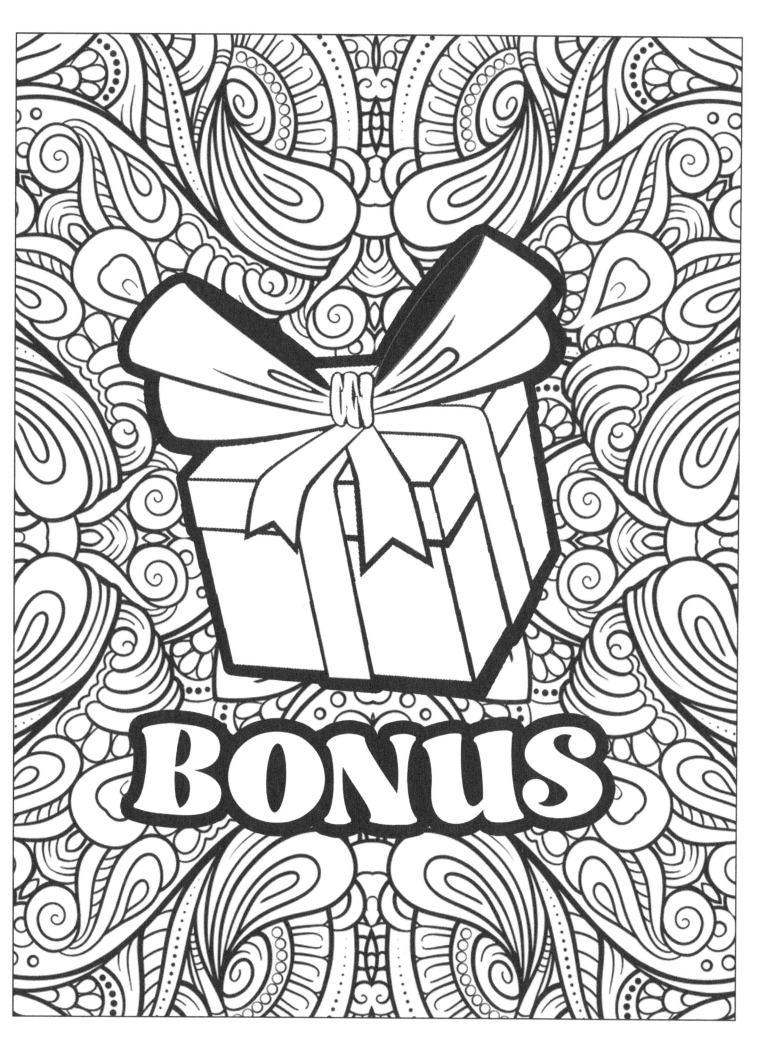

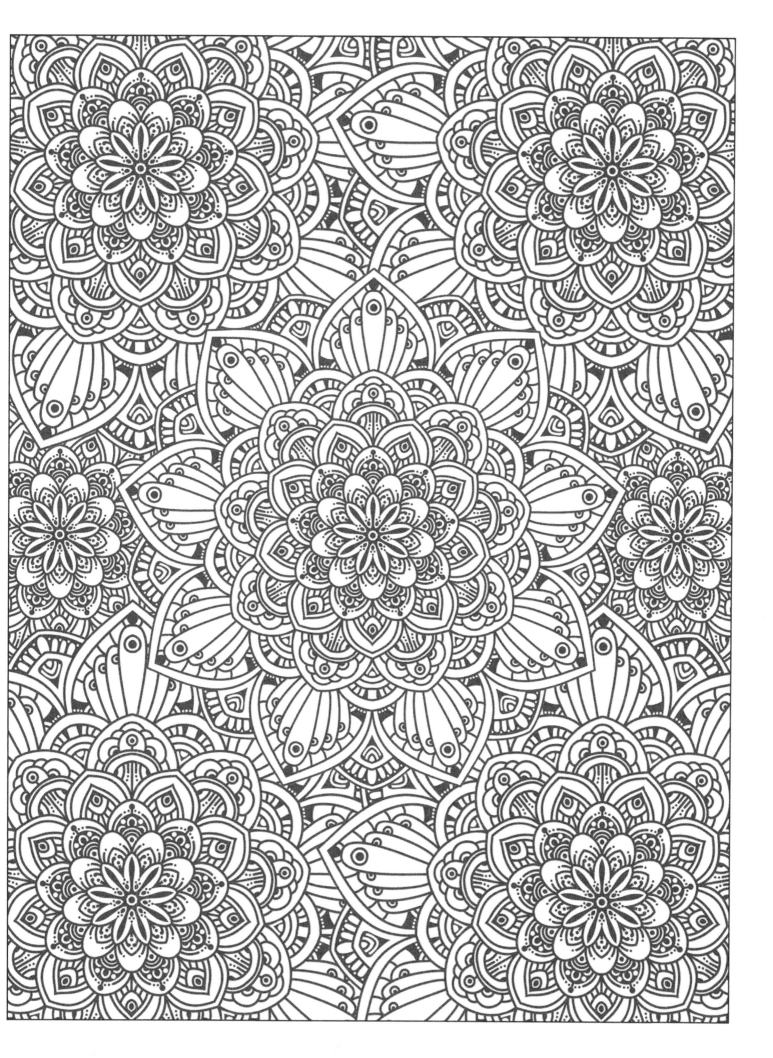

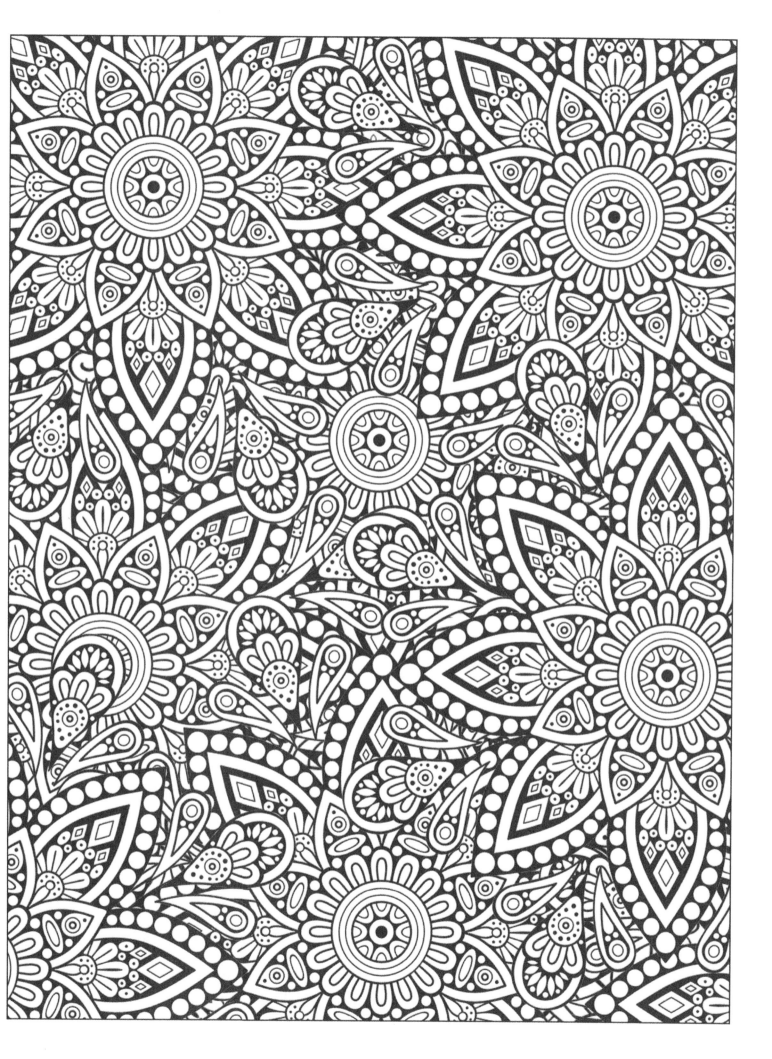

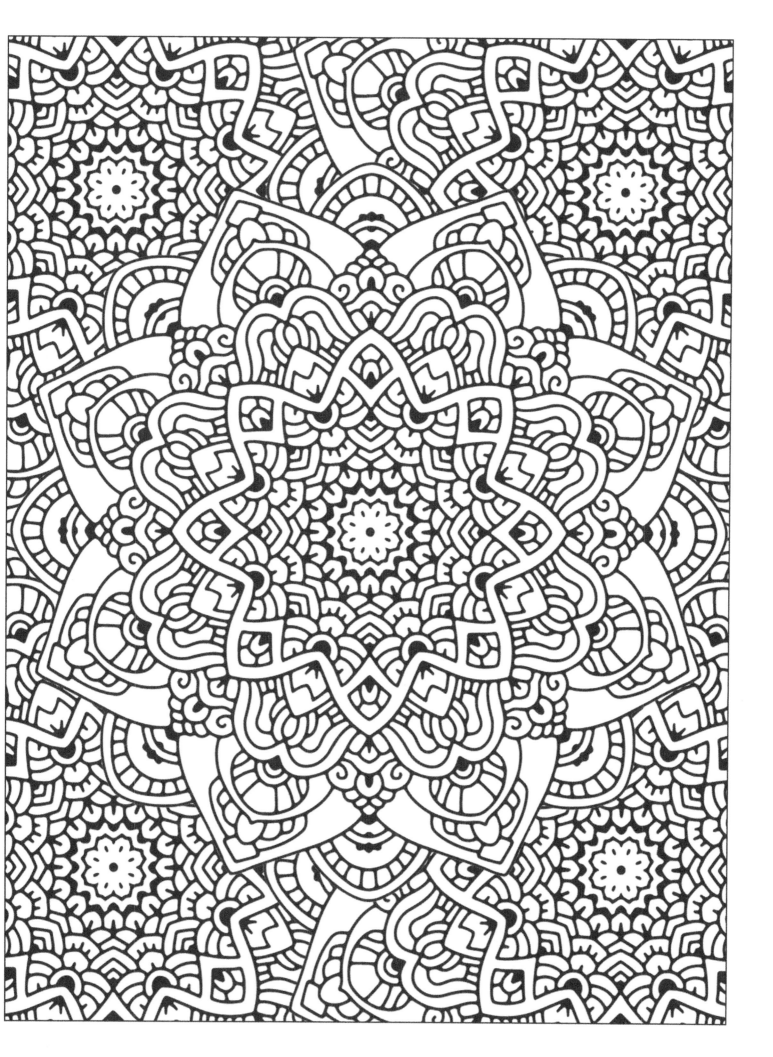

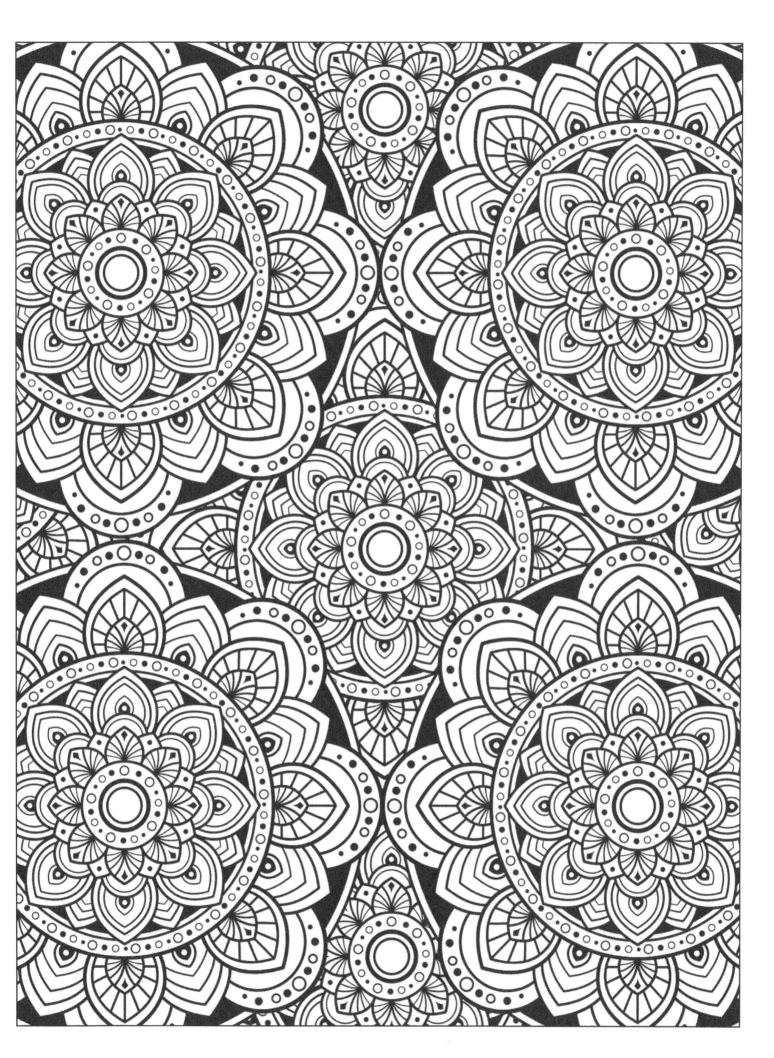

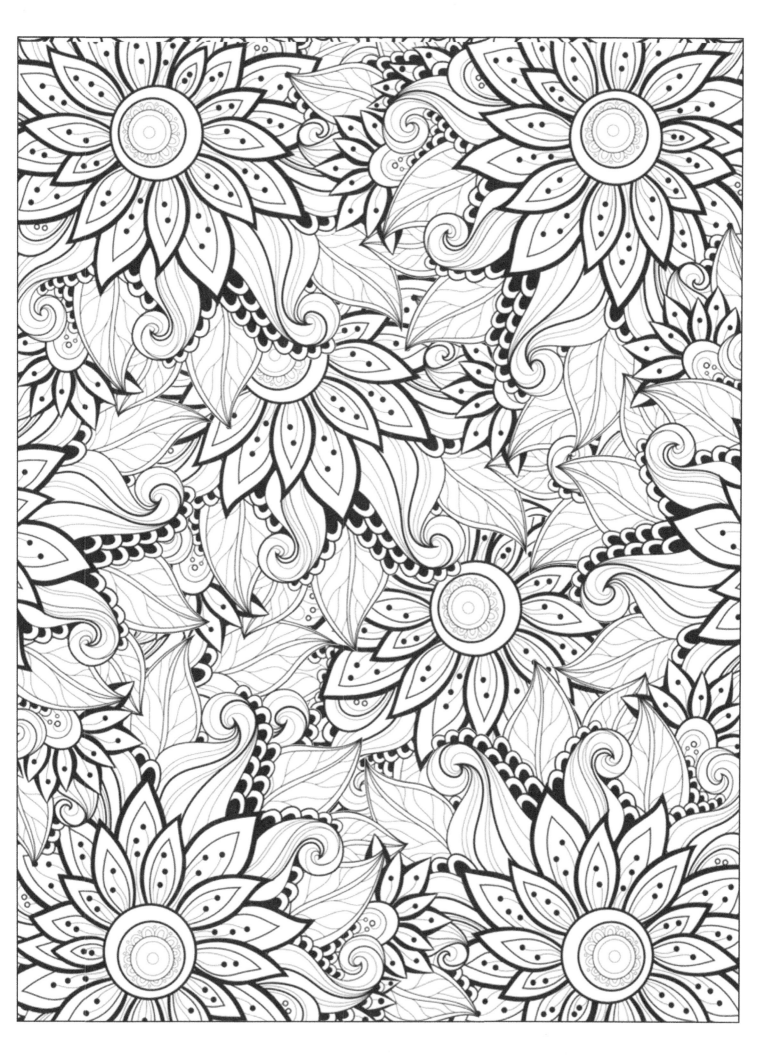

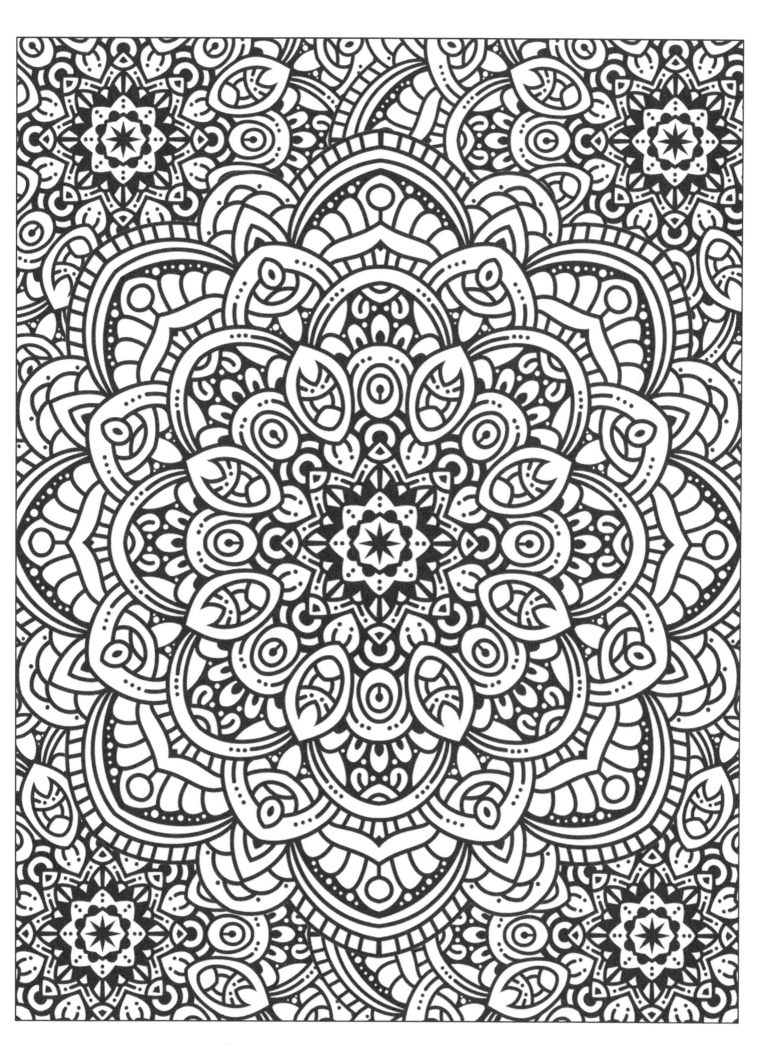

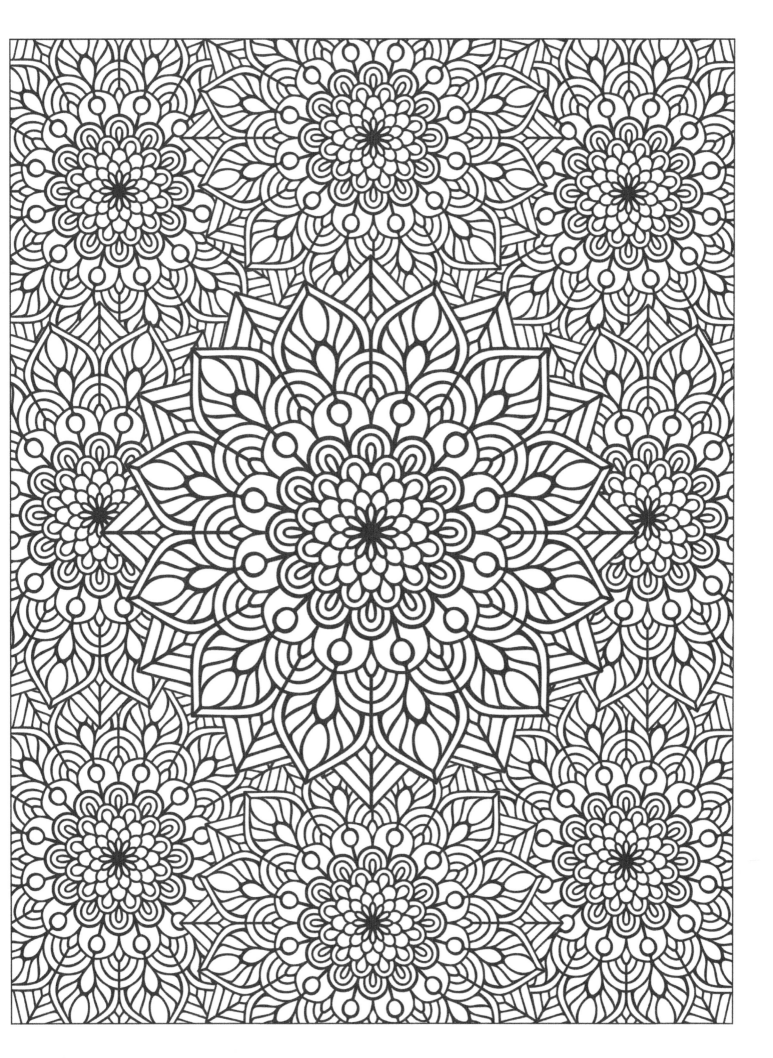

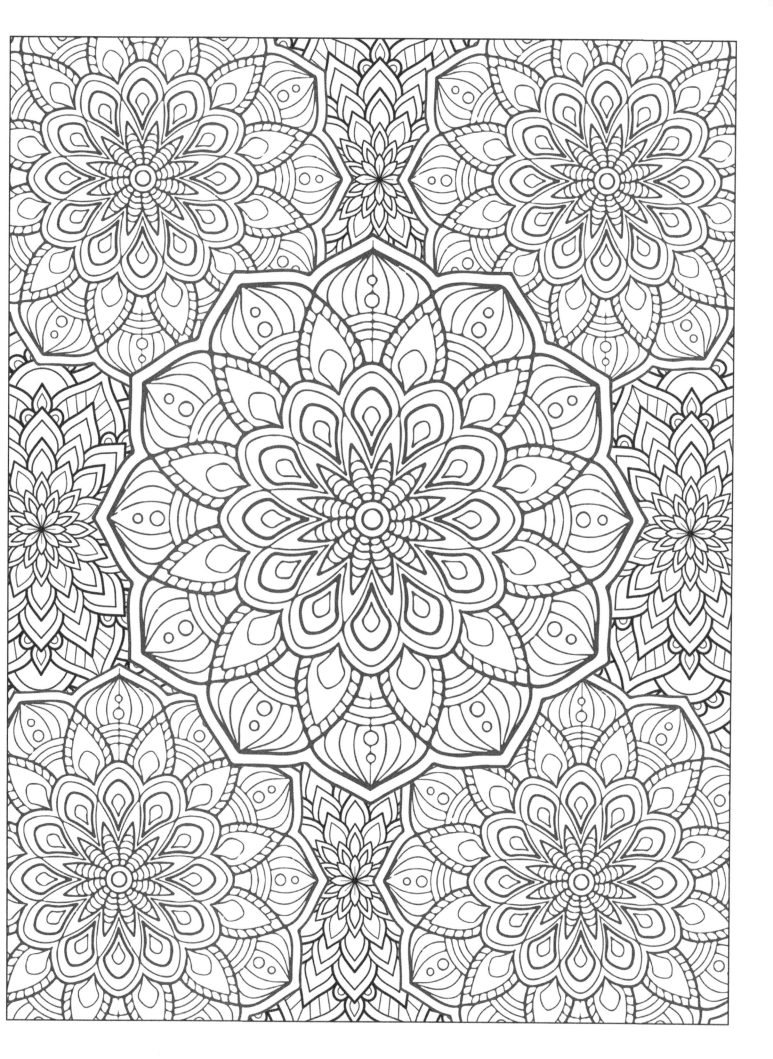

Made in the USA
Middletown, DE
12 March 2025

72602063R00037